Fitness and Nutrition

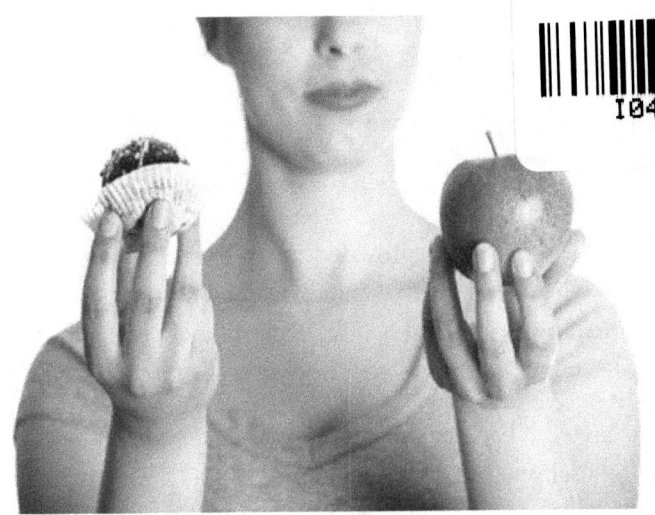

Health Learning Series

M. Usman

Mendon Cottage Books

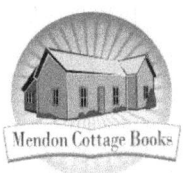

JD-Biz Publishing

Disclaimer

The information is this book is provided for informational purposes only. It is not intended to be used and medical advice or a substitute for proper medical treatment by a qualified health care provider. The information is believed to be accurate as presented based on research by the author.

The contents have not been evaluated by the U.S. Food and Drug Administration or any other Government or Health Organization and the contents in this book are not to be used to treat cure or prevent disease.

The author or publisher is not responsible for the use or safety of any diet, procedure, or treatment mentioned in this book. The author or publisher is not responsible for errors or omissions that may exist.

Warning

The Book is for informational purposes only and before taking on any diet, treatment, or medical procedure, it is recommended to consult with your primary health care provider.

Our books are available at

1. Amazon.com
2. Barnes and Noble
3. Itunes
4. Kobo
5. Smashwords
6. Google Play Books

Table of Contents

Preface

There is nothing elusive about staying fit. The problem is that many people are simply unaware of what must be done to maintain good health. Our poor lifestyles are the roadblocks keeping us from achieving optimum fitness.

One-half of the problem has to do with our diets that are mostly filled with junk. Unfortunately, eating like this keeps our fitness goals from being nothing more than dreams. This type of food has no nutritional value and is usually filled with more calories than we need.

Additionally, we have come to love a sedentary lifestyle, and much of our time is spent watching TV or surfing the internet.

But, for your information, poor nutrition and an inactive lifestyle are the two things making us this way. Thanks to these two, the majority of us are now sick. But, most importantly, there is no way anyone can stay fit living this way.

In this book, you will learn the reason why eating healthy foods is the answer to staying fit. Furthermore, we will look at the need for physical activity and its link to nutrition.

You will also discover the type of foods you should eat and the ones you should avoid. There are a lot of tips on exercising, staying motivated, and more.

So without wasting any more time, begin reading this book. I am sure you will find it helpful.

Chapter # 1: What Is Nutrition?

Nutrition is one of those words you always think you know meaning of until someone asks what it is. The problem is that we use the word interchangeably, leaving others clueless to its actual meaning. But, it's not supposed to be that way. This chapter will give you the simplest meaning of this word.

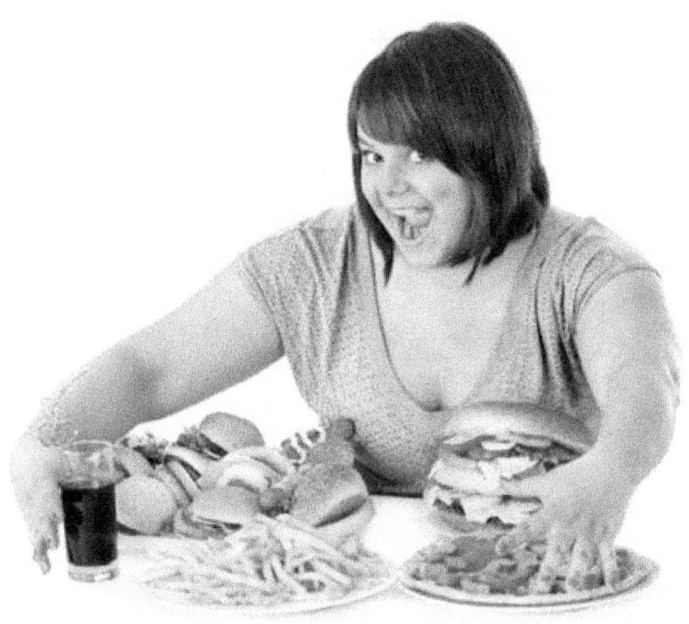

Defining Nutrition

Simply put, it's the supply of essential materials for giving life to the body. By materials, I'm referring to food. Although you might also consider heat, air, and other things as crucial for life, nutrition only focuses on food.

Food is much like fuel. Even the best car in the world is nothing without gas. The same is true for you, if you do not get the necessary nutrients. These are what keep our cells alive, and without them, we wouldn't move, think, or do anything.

Age, strength, or gender does not matter – we all need nutrients to live.

What to Eat

Beginners might not exactly know the foods they should be eating. Furthermore, many are uninformed about the functions of different nutrients in the body. In this chapter, you will learn all about this.

Nutrients are divided into two groups: macronutrients and micronutrients.

Macronutrients are needed by the body in large amounts, while micronutrients are the complete opposite. However, that doesn't mean micronutrients are not important. As a matter of fact, being deficient in them can be disastrous.

Macronutrients

There are only 3 of these: Carbohydrates, Proteins, and Fats. Let's look at them in detail.

Carbohydrates

Carbohydrates are the main source of energy. Fats and proteins come second and third, respectively. For every gram of carbohydrates, you get 4 calories. The recommendation is to have 45 – 65% of this nutrient in your diet.

Some sources of this include fruits, vegetables, bread, rice, pasta, etc.

Proteins

This is another important nutrient you cannot live without. It builds and repairs muscles. In cases where there are no carbohydrates or fats, it may also be used to provide energy. But, when it gets to that, it's a dangerous situation. The body is literally eating itself.

Proteins are also used in the making of enzymes and hormones.

Depending in several factors, the recommendation is to have 10 – 35% of this nutrient in your diet. Some of the best sources include eggs, beans, low-fat meat, nuts, milk, chicken, etc.

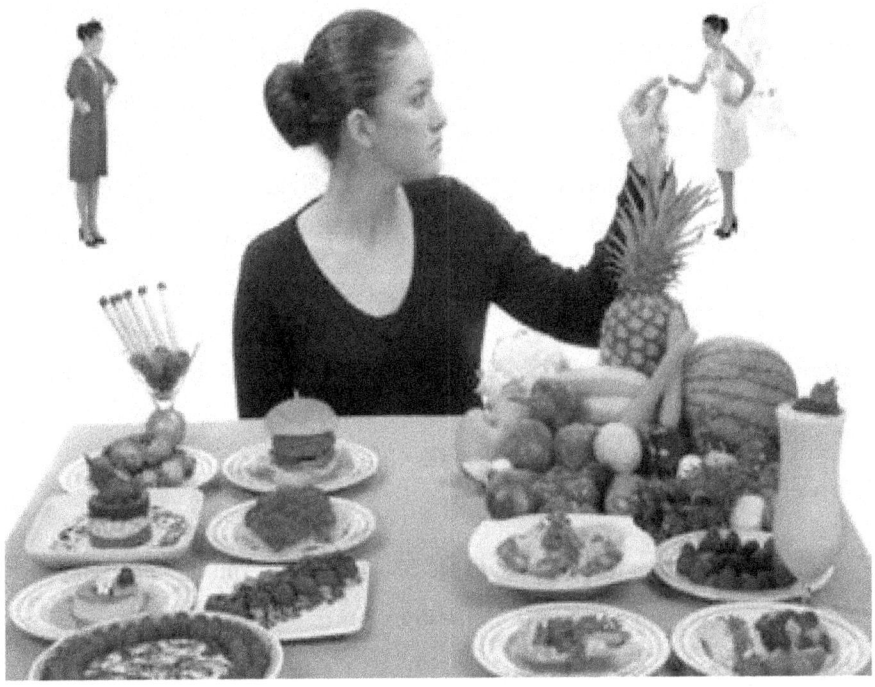

Fats

You might have heard that fats are bad for your health, but this is not necessarily so. There are some fats that are good for your body.

Apart from providing energy, fats are also responsible for increasing the absorption of fat-soluble vitamins. Besides that, they also help keep the body warm.

You are supposed to have about 20% fat in your diet. For every gram of this nutrient, you get 9 calories. Some of the best sources are fish, walnuts, vegetable based oils, olive oil, avocados, etc.

You should focus on getting unsaturated fats, as these are the healthier type. Saturated and Trans fats are the ones you should avoid.

Micronutrients

As stated previously, these are needed in small quantities, and there are only two of them:

Vitamins: These have a range of functions in the body, and they come from different foods. They can be used to boost immunity, improve vision, and other life important functions. Some of the vitamins include A, B, C, D, etc.

Minerals: These are also important in the normal functionality of the body. They include zinc, magnesium, potassium, phosphorous, iron, etc.

Water

A good proportion of our body is made up of liquids. And having it in short supply can leave you feeling tired, inhibit your cognitive abilities, and more.

In conclusion, it's true that you have the freedom to eat what you want. However, you should limit your choices to only what is deemed healthy. For example, Trans and Saturated fats, together with sugary foods, should not find their way into your mouth.

Chapter # 2: The Link between Fitness and Nutrition

Fitness and nutrition go hand in hand. There is no way you can successfully have one without the other; hence, the importance of following good nutrition guidelines. That will be the only key to realizing your fitness goals.

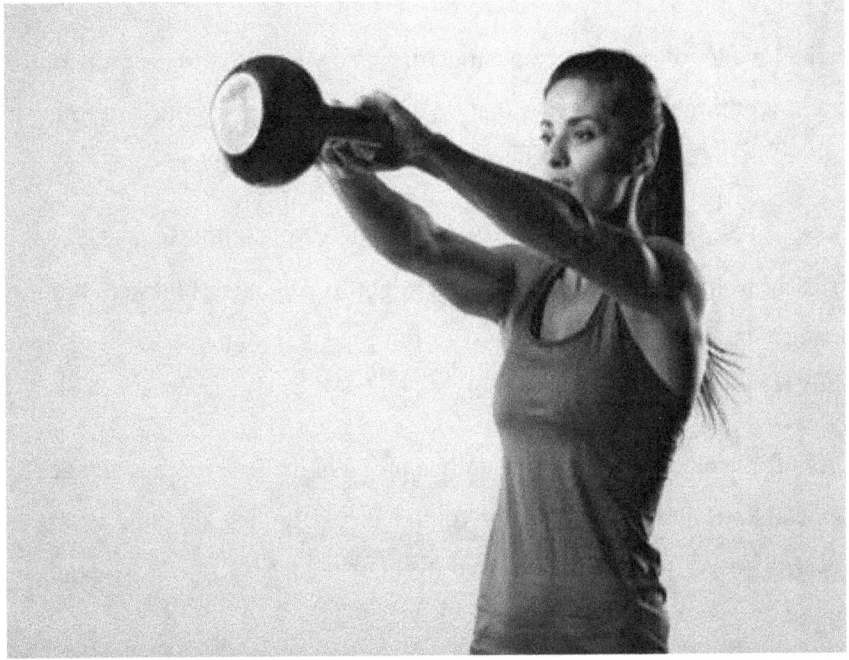

Reasons for taking part in a fitness program vary among individuals. Here are a few:

- ***Wanting to Improve Appearance***: For women, the goal is to slim down like someone on a magazine. On the other hand, men want muscle.

- ***Lose Weight***: Those who are overweight might start working out to shed some pounds after learning the negative effects of their condition.

- ***Stay Fit***: Everybody wants to have a body capable of doing just about anything. The only way to achieve that is through exercising.

- ***Improve Mood:*** Physical activity improves your mood by reducing stress and depression.

There are a lot of benefits you can get from staying fit. However, the most important thing is to realize is that no matter how intense your workout, you will only see the benefits with proper nutrition.

Energy: Food provides the body with energy. Without this, you are no different from a car with no fuel. You might force yourself through the exercise, but you will not realize your full potential. In the worst cases, you won't be able to even raise a finger.

Loss of muscle mass: This is usually a problem that increases with age. It can lead to disability, minimizing your chances of doing anything to stay fit. But with proper nutrition, you can prevent or reduce the rate at which this happens.

Taking time for the body to heal: Exercising destroys muscles, and when you eat, they are repaired, leading to growth and a boost in strength. But, without a proper diet, you will not see any of those benefits.

Muscle Fatigue: Although water is not a nutrient per se, it's still one thing you should get enough of. Depriving yourself of it can backfire, as our bodies are largely made up of liquids. And, during physical activity, a good amount of this is used up. If not replaced, it can lead to muscle fatigue.

Missed Menstruation: For other women, poor nutrition can lead to the missing of their period.

Weak Immune System: Because you do not get all the necessary nutrients with improper nutrition, your immunity may become weak and susceptible to attack.

However, when you have a good diet in place, all these problems will not be present. You will be able to work out as much as you want, without burning your fuel reserves. In the end, achieving your fitness goals will be easy.

Chapter # 3: How the Body Uses Energy

As someone who works out and eats the right foods to stay fit, you will need to understand how the body uses energy. After all, it's what keeps us alive.

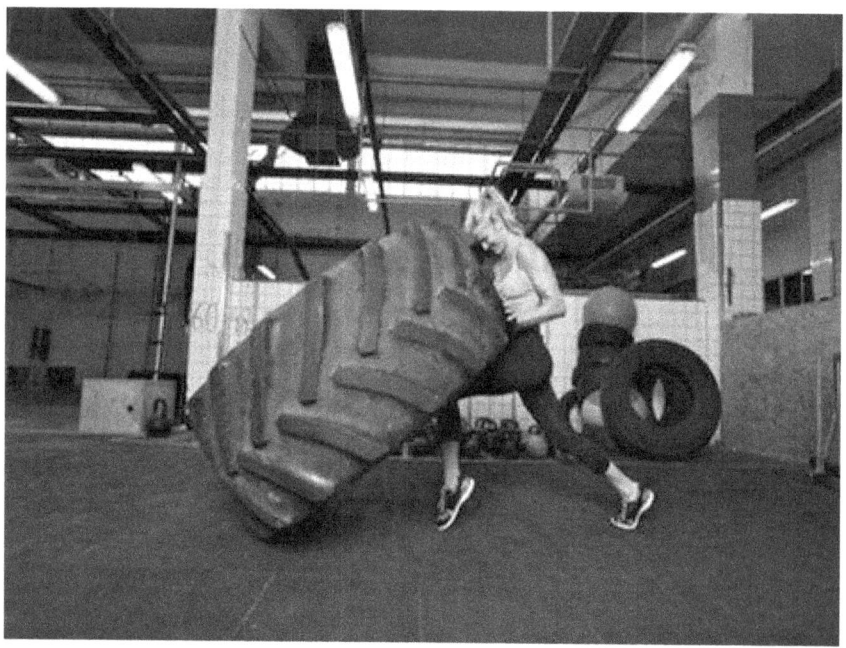

Science clearly dictates that energy cannot be made. So, the body must get it from somewhere else, and this source happens to be the food we eat daily (bread, pasta, meat, fruit, etc.).

How the Process Works

When we chew the food, it breaks down, and this is normally the start of digestion. By the time it reaches the stomach, acids and other enzymes digest it even further. For carbohydrates, the result is a sugar called glucose.

This is then absorbed into the bloodstream. Beta cells, which are sensitive to an increase in glucose, then order the pancreas to start producing insulin.

Insulin is a hormone that tells cells to absorb the glucose in the blood, thereby bringing its levels down. When glucose is inside the cells, it's used for energy or stored for later use.

Since the level of sugar has decreased, the pancreas will reduce the production of insulin, so blood sugar levels return to normal.

Problems with Eating Sugary Foods

If you have a sweet tooth, know that it's dangerous for your health. Constantly eating foods that are high in sugar, forces your body to produce insulin all the time. Making it worse, these foods leave you feeling empty in just a few hours, so you will likely eat more.

With insulin levels high all the time, you can end up with a condition known as insulin resistance. This may result in Type 1 Diabetes.

With this condition, your body does not produce insulin or fails to make good use of the available insulin. Therefore, your cells will have a hard time absorbing the glucose in your blood. In the end, you will find yourself feeling weak all the time. And, if you were thinking of a workout, you would certainly not have the energy for it.

When you eat healthy foods, those low in sugar and high in fiber, you can be spared from those issues. You will have energy to do your workouts and stay fit. Additionally, since you will be eating all the needed nutrients, your immunity and overall healthy will improve.

Chapter # 4: Nutritional Guidelines

The purpose of these guidelines is to educate you on the necessity of adopting a good diet and staying active. You will learn how to make healthy food choices, and, at the same time, halt the behaviors that can destroy your life.

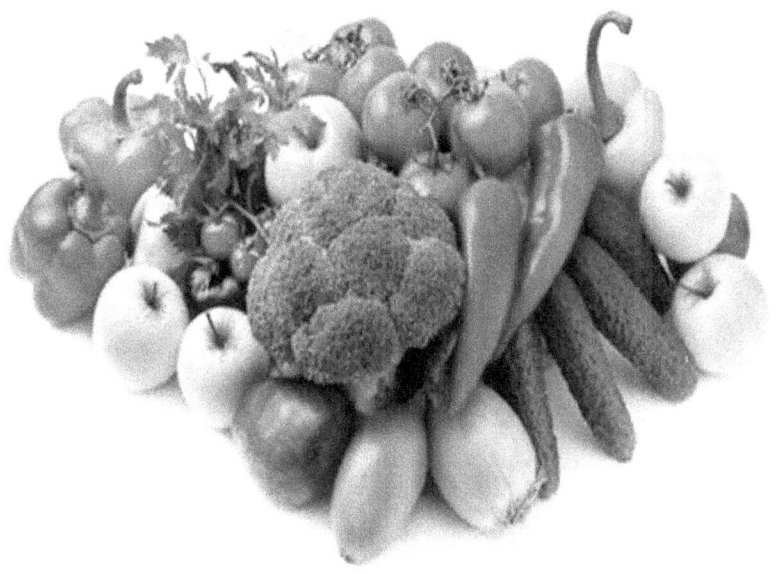

For most of us, sticking to a single diet can be a nightmare, and it's understandable. Eating the same things daily is boring. But it is not meant to be that way. Staying healthy does not make you a slave. You still need to have autonomy to eat and move the way you want to, as long as your choices are healthy ones.

Here are the guidelines:

- ***Consume a Variety of Nutritious Foods***: You should make an effort to eat food from all the groups. That will eliminate the possibility of missing some nutrients. All the nutrients we talked about earlier are important, and being deficient in them can have life-threatening consequences.

- *Avoid Sugars*: Despite being pleasing to the taste buds, there is nothing good about too much sugar. It makes you gain weight and leads to other undesirable results.

- *Reduce Salt Intake*: Too much of this can lead to high blood pressure, heart failure, or heart attack.

- *Limit Alcohol Intake*: Men should aim for 2 bottles of beer per day while women should keep it at 1.

- *Limit Saturated and Trans Fats*: These are unhealthy and can cause mayhem to your healthy. So, by all means, avoid them like the plague. Unsaturated fats are the ones you should be eating.

- *Don't Forget Fiber:* From making you feel full to aiding in digestion and more, fiber is one thing you should have enough of in your diet.

- *Clean Hands, Food, and Food Contact Surfaces:* These could be harboring dangerous germs. If allowed into your body, you could end up getting sick.

- *Limit Cholesterol*: Another thing you do not want in your body is cholesterol. It is dangerous to your health. Before buying food, read the labels, and if it has lots of this, stay away from it.

- ***Control Calorie Intake***: It's easy to get carried away and eat more than you really need. Even if it's healthy foods you are crushing, you could be packing up too many calories. Eat only what you believe is enough to sustain you. Otherwise, you will only increase your body weight.

You should focus on eating lots of fruits, vegetables, lean meats, low-fat milk, fish, whole grains, beans, eggs, and other healthy foods.

Chapter # 5: Activity-Specific Nutrition

Before starting with everything, it's crucial to be clear of your goals. The same is true if you are adopting a nutrition plan. Are you trying to lose weight? Or is it muscle you are trying to build? Perhaps you just want to be fit?

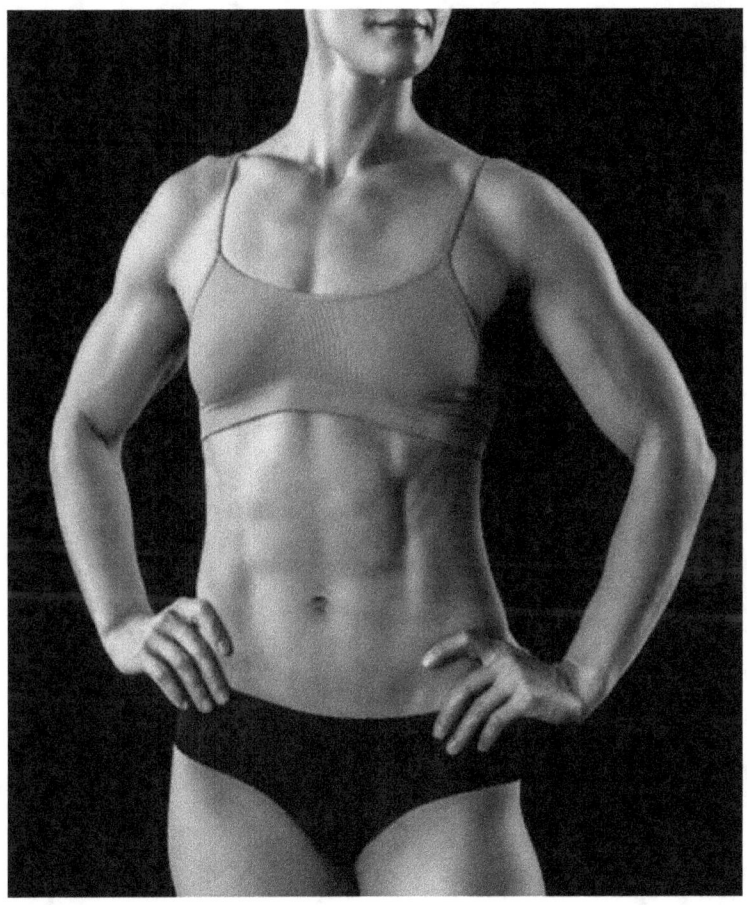

Your answers to these questions will determine what you will eat, but this does not mean you will get back to eating junk. Rather, it will be the same food with emphasis on certain nutrients.

Losing Weight

If trying to get rid of some pounds, you will need to reduce your calorie intake. This is possible by using more calories that you consume. Normally, you should create a 500 calorie deficit daily.

Sugars and other unhealthy fats should not be present in your diet. As a rule of thumb, eat real food. That means anything that has undergone heavy processing should not end up in mouth.

Another thing to watch out for is the reward after exercise. Specifically, do not bring an energy drink or any type of food to the gym. A 30-minute workout doesn't need this. You will only add back the calories you just finished burning.

Furthermore, you will need to limit your snacks between meals.

Body Building

If you are trying to gain muscle, the situation is much different. Although you are also bound to eating only healthy foods, the way you eat it will differ from someone losing weight.

Since bodybuilding workouts break your body, you will need to eat accordingly to repair your muscles. You will find yourself eating more proteins than ever before. Additionally, you may need to eat more often.

Athletes

If you are an athlete, you will need even more food. But, unlike those losing weight or building muscle, the nutritional focus will differ. Some training sessions can last for more than 90 minutes, requiring lots of energy. But that is no license to eat as much as your stomach can handle. You will still need to eat only what you think is necessary.

As you can see, what you eat largely depends on how active you are. If you are not sure about what you will need to eat, talk to someone experienced to help you.

If you an average Joe, there is nothing special you need. Watch your food choices, your portion sizes, and do some physical activity. You will maintain a healthy weight and be fit at that same time.

Chapter # 6: Vegan Nutrition

The thought of fitness and vegan nutrition may seem like a journey down a river. And honestly, this is no surprise at all. A diet with no meat, milk, eggs, or many other foods, doesn't sound so promising. And, if you are a bodybuilder or an athlete, you might not believe it's even possible.

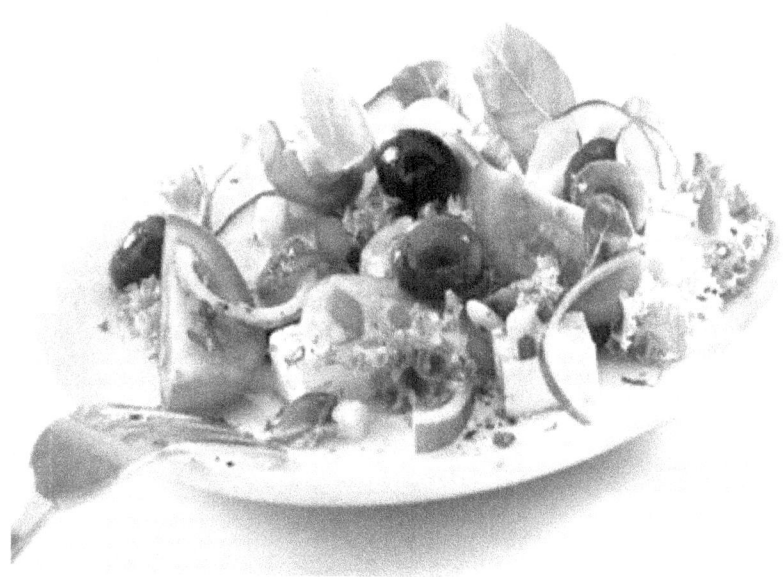

Nevertheless, vegan nutrition and fitness are very feasible. While you are limited in terms of what you can eat, it's still possible to get all the necessary nutrients. It's true that the foods in this diet might not provide all the recommended quantities of nutrients, but you can take supplements to make up for it.

However, many people are under the impression that going vegetarian leaves you immune to the dangers of foods. If you are careless, you could be eating lots of calories and gain weight in the end. This is also the case if you are eating a lot of sugar.

If you also have a lot of processed foods, be mindful of the ingredients in the food. A label saying it's healthy doesn't really mean it is. Some of the foods are high in sodium, which is also very dangerous in itself.

If you have chosen to take this route, here are some foods with the nutrients you need:

Protein: If you are not a vegan, you have a whole lot of foods at your disposal. But, for vegans, there is not much room for treating your taste buds. Some foods with protein include soy foods, nuts, seeds, whole grains, etc.

Fats and Oils: You should focus on eating lots of healthful oils from olive, canola, avocado, walnuts, hemp seeds, etc.

Calcium: Some sources of this include broccoli, green leafy vegetables, almonds, Brazil nuts, chickpeas, sesame seeds, etc.

Iron: Sources include watermelons, whole grains, spinach, cereals, green leafy vegetables, and many more.

Other foods include bananas, strawberries, mushrooms, peanuts, oranges, yeast, molasses, carrots, brown rice, tomatoes, and cabbage.

Chapter # 7: Reading Food Labels

A great proportion of our diet is made up of packaged foods. Unless you are willing to start your own farm and produce your own food, learning to read food labels is a skill you should have. With that, you will be able to make the best food choices.

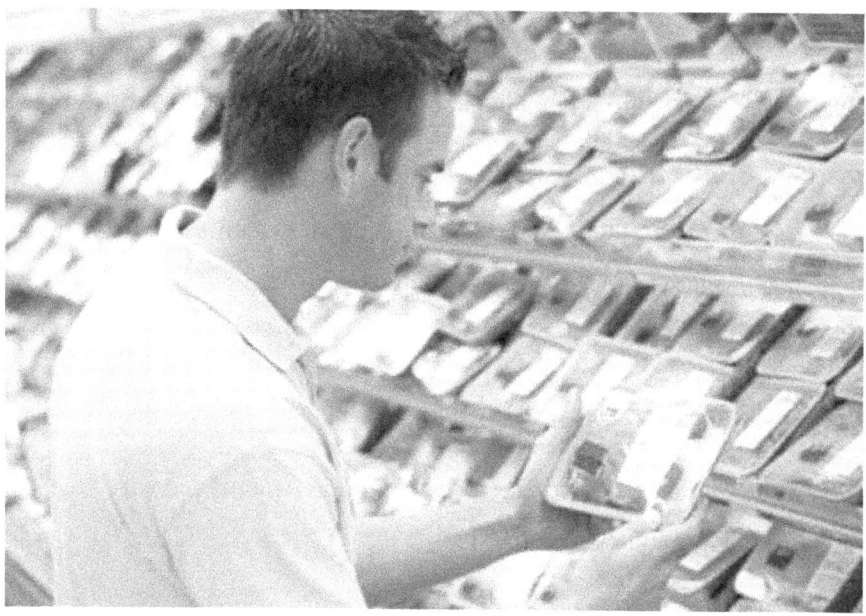

Most of us only see a range of meaningless numbers when looking at the Nutrition Information Panel (NIP). Actually, many give up in frustration and never waste their time looking at the NIP again. But, if you only knew how to read it, you would be shocked to discover that what you eat may not be so healthy.

It's a requirement for every manufacturer to have the NIP on all their foods. This indicates the content of energy, protein, fat, carbohydrates, sugar, sodium, and other important nutrients.

Usually, there are two columns. One shows values per serving and the other indicates values per 100 grams.

You use the first column when figuring out a number of nutrients you will consume in a single serving. For example, drinking a bottle of juice with two servings will mean you will need to double the values in the Per Serving column.

The Per 100 grams column is useful when comparing two or more foods. With this, you can tell which food has more calories, sodium, fats, and other nutrients. If it's a drink in question, this information usually comes per 100ml.

Here are some things to remember when looking at the NIP:

Fat: You should limit your intake of Saturated and Trans fats. On the NIP, go for food with less than 2g of saturated fat per 100g. As for total fat, it should be less than 10g per 100g

Fiber: Fiber is important in making you feel full and reducing the chances of constipation. For every 100g, there should be more than 6g of fiber.

Sodium: This is another thing you should limit in intake. So, choose foods with less than 120mg of sodium per 100g. If the NIP shows more than 600mg per 100g, you are looking at a food with high levels of this mineral

Sugar: This is famous for all the wrong reasons. So for every 100g, make sure you have less than 10g of it.

Since comparing foods in a shop can take time, focus on analyzing two or three foods at a time. Additionally, don't forget to bring your reading glasses if you have eye problems.

Chapter # 8: Tips for Exercising

Some level of physical activity is needed in order to stay fit. This must be paired with good nutrition to achieve the best results. Workouts can range from walking to lifting weights. Mainly, your fitness goals will determine the type of exercise you will do.

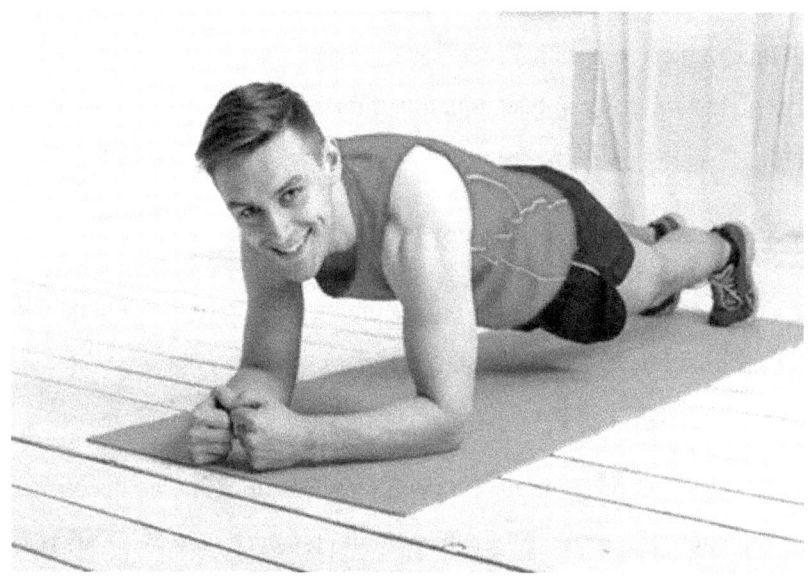

Due to lack of knowledge, many miss important elements that can determine the chances of a successful workout. This chapter will introduce you to some tips you should always keep in mind.

Warming Up

Before beginning any exercise, you always need to warm up. Five to ten minutes is all you need to get started. The warm-up should not be intense, as you are just trying to get your body ready for the exercises that are to follow.

For starters, jogging, dancing, walking, and other low-intensity exercises will do just fine.

The Exercise

When the body is ready, you can move on to the main workout. There are a range of aerobic and anaerobic exercises you can do. This includes push-ups, running, weight lifting, jump ropes, etc.

You should aim for at least 30 minutes of moderate intensity exercises 5 times a week. If doing high-intensity workouts, you can get away with 20 minutes per day.

A major mistake many commit is doing the same workout every time. Your muscles adapt to the exercise, making it less effective. Furthermore, some muscles do not get the attention they need. So if you were trying to build strength all over your body, this would remain a dream.

As a solution, combine cardio and anaerobic exercises in your workouts. Another thing you should look out for is over-exercising. If your body is aching all the time, and you can't even finish a workout, you could be abusing yourself. And this is not good for you.

Stretching

There are disagreements on whether you should stretch after or before a workout. Studies have failed to prove that stretching before a workout increases performance. However, doing it after you have finished exercising does make your body feel flexible.

Time of Exercise

Some believe in exercising in the morning while others swear to exercising in the evening. We are all different and we live different lives. Try doing both and decide which of the two serves you best.

If you have a condition that prevents you from exercising, talk to your doctor. He might be able to figure out some physical activity suitable for your condition. A sedentary lifestyle does not help make you fit.

Chapter # 9: Tips for Staying Motivated

Time and again, many set themselves on a road to fitness only to realize they are drifting back to unhealthy lifestyles. Owing to this, they continue gaining weight, being plagued by diseases, and a whole lot of other issues.

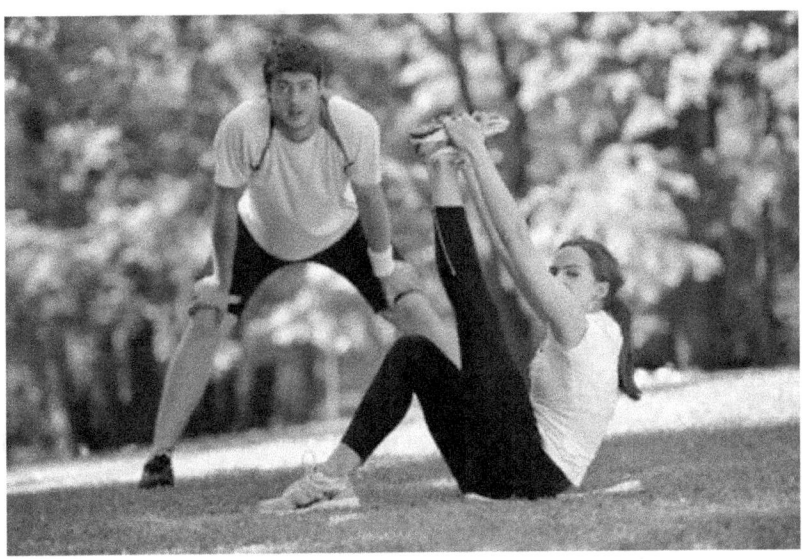

But this isn't something to beat yourself down for. Staying on a diet or fitness program is easier said than done. Eating the same things daily can numb your taste buds, and there are always good excuses for skipping a workout.

From experience, these problems are usually present when you are just getting started. Once you have been at it for a year or more, living a healthy lifestyle becomes easier. Actually, there will be no difference between brushing your teeth every morning and going for a run every night.

Here are the tips to keep you motivated:

Have a Workout Buddy: When just starting out, it's difficult to work out on your own. You will always find a better excuse for shifting your workout to another day. But, with a workout buddy, you will always feel accountable to someone. Your buddy will push you when you don't feel like moving.

If you can, join a CrossFit gym near you. You will be motivated by the team spirit that's always there.

Set Goals: If you had billions of dollars, you certainly wouldn't be bothering yourself getting up every morning to get to work. That's because you would have no valid reason to work. But, you get up every day because you have to feed the family, buy gas, and more. Your goal is to make money at the end of every month.

With the same analogy, you can set goals for your healthy lifestyle. Are you trying to lose weight? Is it muscle you want? Having a goal will keep focused on doing what it takes to get the results. Just make sure your goals are achievable and measurable.

Record Results: Not knowing or overlooking the small gains you have made is what forces many to give up too early. But, if you were to record your results, you would be able to look back and take pride in your achievements.

Start Slow: Another mistake is that many try to hit high notes from the very start. However, this is simply unrealistic. Acknowledge that your muscles are not yet used to such activities. If it's a new diet, understand that it will take time for your body to get used to your new eating habit. So, go slow and build up momentum with time.

Variety: The problem with many diets or exercise routines is that they are so restrictive. They will tell you to only eat A, B, C, and D. Same thing with workouts, as you will be told do 1, 2, and 3. But, this kills the fun you should be having. As a solution, keep varying the foods you eat and never do the same exercise every time. After all, we all know that variety is the spice of life.

Reward Yourself: By that I do not mean you guzzle on an energy drink after your finish your workout. Rather, buy yourself new clothes or shoes for achieving your goal. Be creative and reward yourself in a way you think is best.

Chapter # 10: Avoid Nutritional Deficiencies

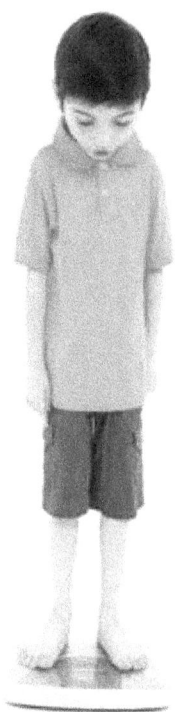

It is possible to go wrong, even when you are living a healthy lifestyle. When just starting out, you need to pay attention and be sure that you are getting all the nutrients you need.

Unfortunately, it's not always easy to know if you are deficient in some. You might see symptoms only to dismiss them for something else. By the time you realize you weren't getting enough of a certain nutrient, the damage may have already been done.

Nutrients you are probably deficient in

From a number of studies, there are a couple of micronutrients lacking in many of us. This is regardless of the fact that most vitamins and minerals are needed in small amounts.

For the macronutrients, it's usually proteins and fats that we don't get enough of. Carbohydrates are almost present in every food, so it's easy to get them in adequate amounts.

Here are the nutrients many are deficient in:

- Vitamin D

- Calcium

- Magnesium

- B vitamins

- Iron

Symptoms of nutrient deficiencies

Since it's micronutrients we are mostly deficient in, seeing the effect right away might not be so easy. Usually, it will take time before you can develop the real symptoms. Here are some things you should be on the lookout for:

- If you are having unexplained fatigue all the time, it might be a sign of some nutritional deficiency.

- Cracking in the corners of the mouth is usually an indication that you do not have enough riboflavin or vitamin C. This might still continue despite your efforts in using lip balm and other solutions.

- Nails that break easily are a great sign that you do not have enough iron.

- Unexplained hair loss or brittle hair is proof that you are not getting enough nutrients.

- Muscles clumps and tingling in the limbs, despite being physically active.

- Lack of appetite all the time.

If you notice these symptoms, visit your doctor. He might run some tests to identify the real cause of your condition.

Solutions to Nutrient Deficiencies

Adopting a healthy diet is not enough in itself. You will need to make sure that you are eating the right amounts of food. Eat too much and you risk consuming a lot of calories. And if you eat too little, you might not get all the nutrients.

Adding to this, you should include a range of foods in your diet. This is very important and cannot be overemphasized. Varying your food sources will make it easy to eat every nutrient.

You should focus on fruits, vegetables, meat, fish, fats, low-fat milk, and other healthy foods. Try to cook most of your meals yourself. And if possible, eat it raw. This is especially true with vegetables. If you are the type that does not like eating vegetables, you can try juicing. You will be getting a concentrated amount of nutrients that way. Juicing uses a lot of vegetables than you would manage to eat in one sitting.

Conclusion

Those are the major issues you needed to know about nutrition and fitness. I hope you found the book useful. As a recap, remember that fitness and nutrition are two interlinked subjects. As I said, you won't have one without the other.

It is crucial that you keep a close eye on what you eat. Remember that you are what you eat. If you want to be healthy, make healthy food choices. Besides that, always make time for some physical activity. Just 30 minutes, or even less, per day is all you need to burn some calories. That will keep your body strong and you will stay fit for your entire life.

Making it even better, you will be able to maintain a healthy weight and avoid diseases associated with obesity.

At first, you might think it will be hard to just give up on food you have loved all these years. But, remember that junk food does not contribute to your health in any way. You will only gain weight and endanger your own immunity in the process. Realize that change is the last option you have got.

With that, I hope you will start making healthy food choices and living an active life. A sedentary lifestyle and poor nutrition do not help. Avoid these two at all cost.

Author Bio

Muhammad Usman is a distinguished medical graduate of Allama Iqbal medical college (AIMC). He is a professional writer who has been in the field for more than 4 years. During this time he has produced 10,000+ articles, blogs, and eBooks on various niches related to diseases, health, fitness, nutrition, and well-being. He is a regular contributor to several journals related to medicine and surgery. He is the editor of several journals and newspapers.

Check out some of the other JD-Biz Publishing books

Gardening Series on Amazon

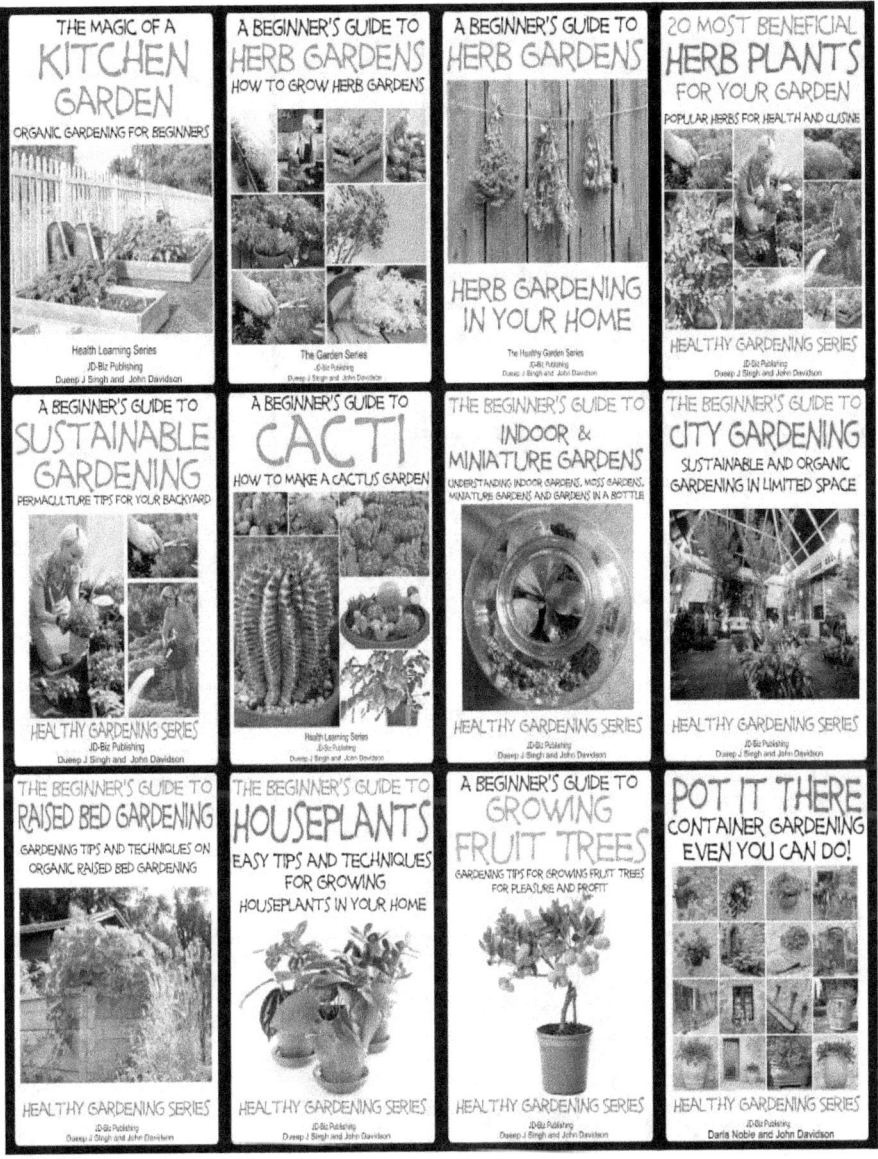

Health Learning Series

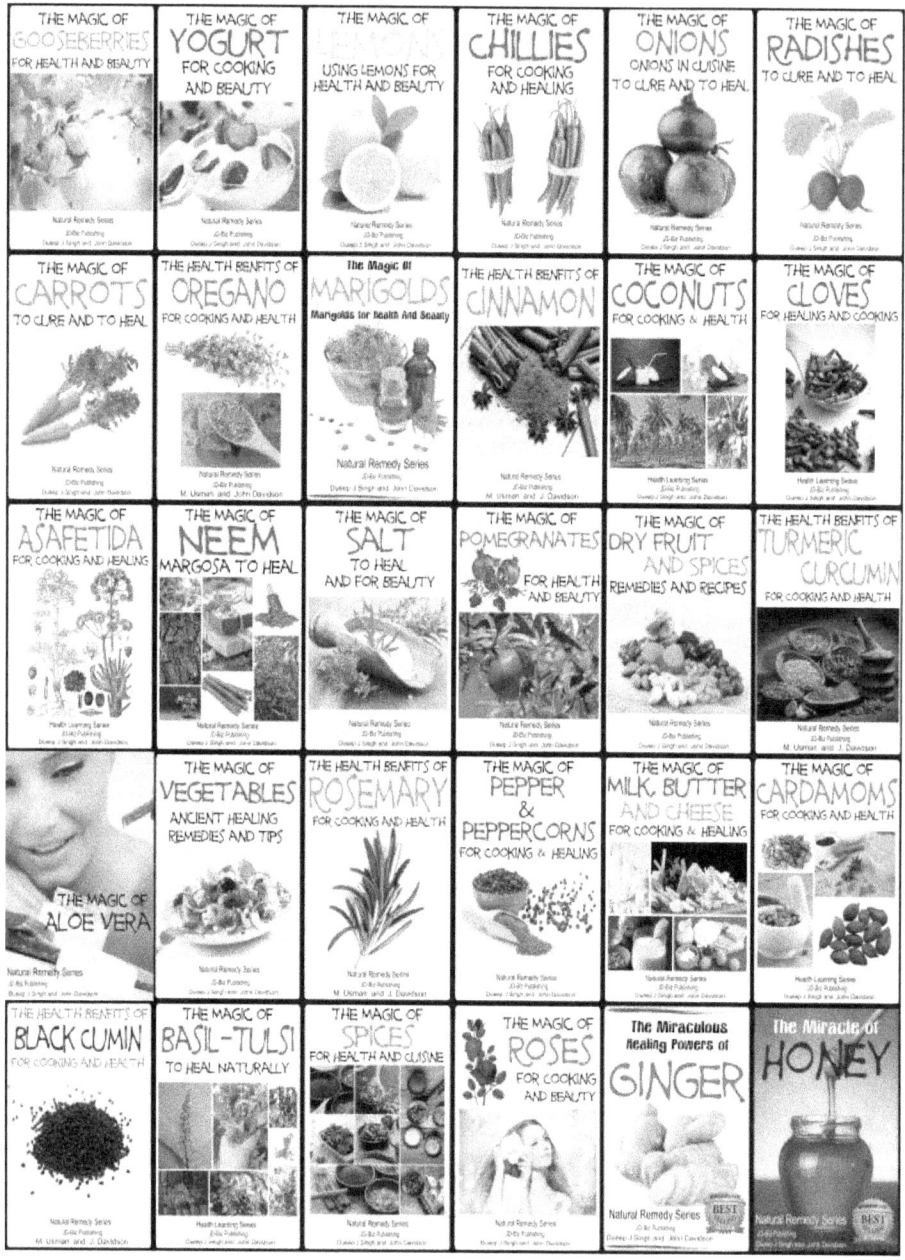

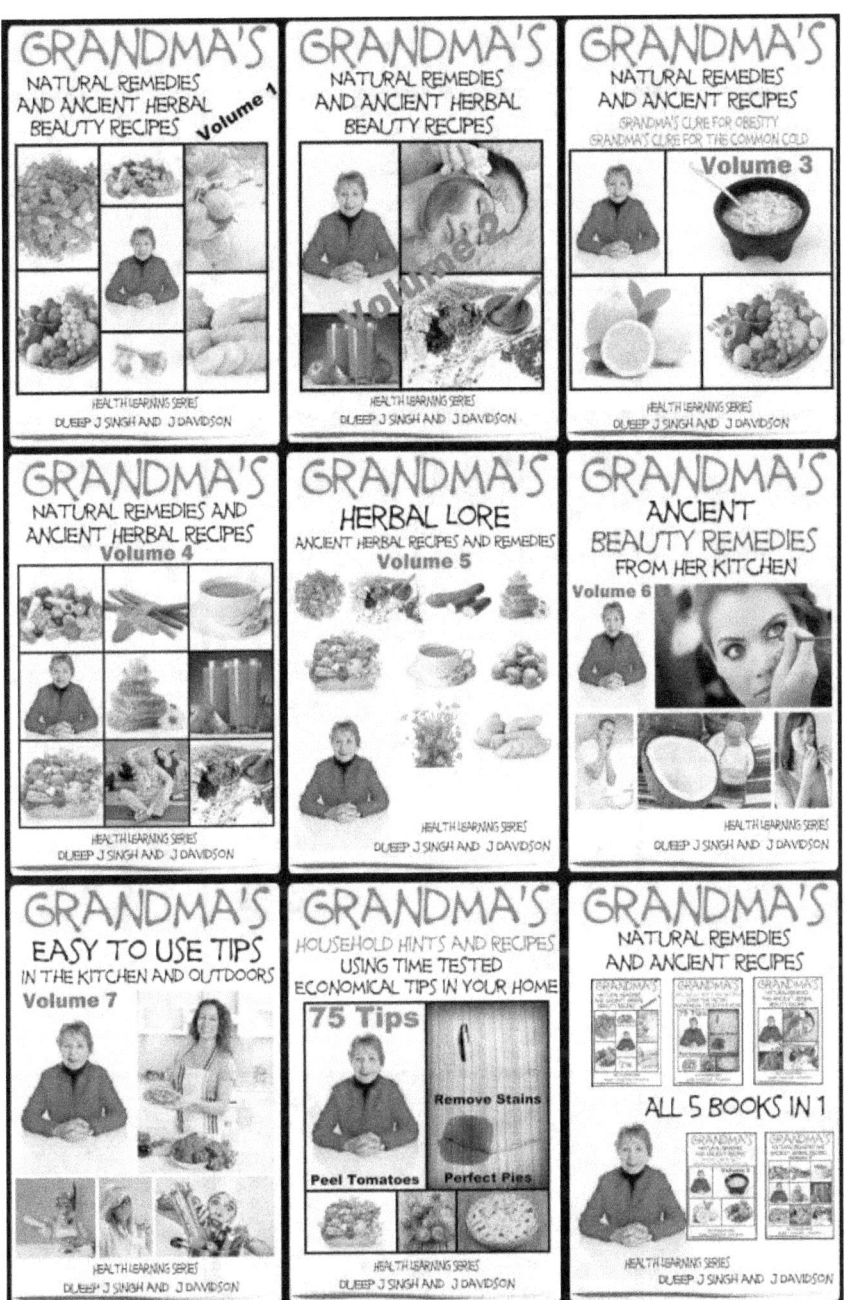

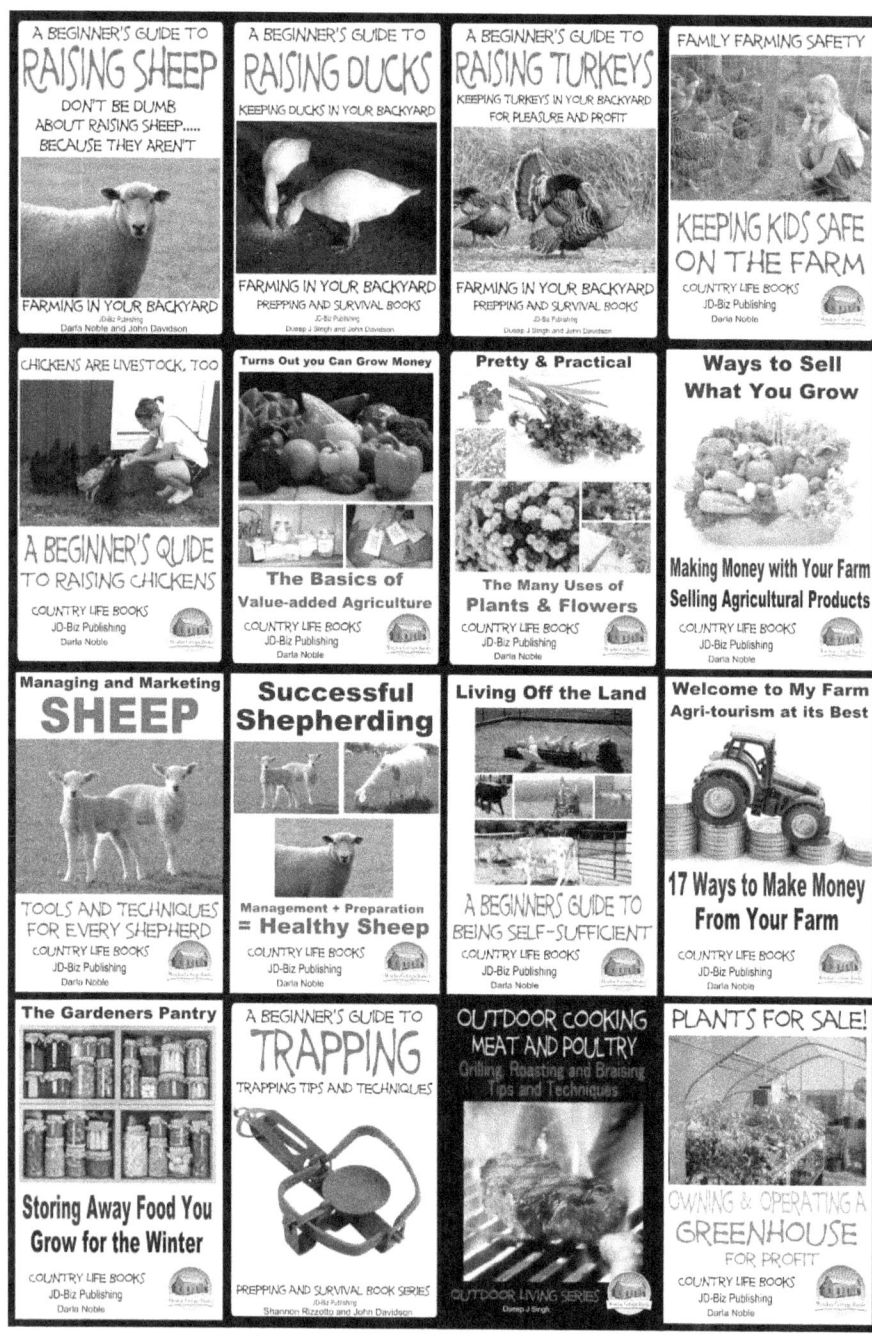

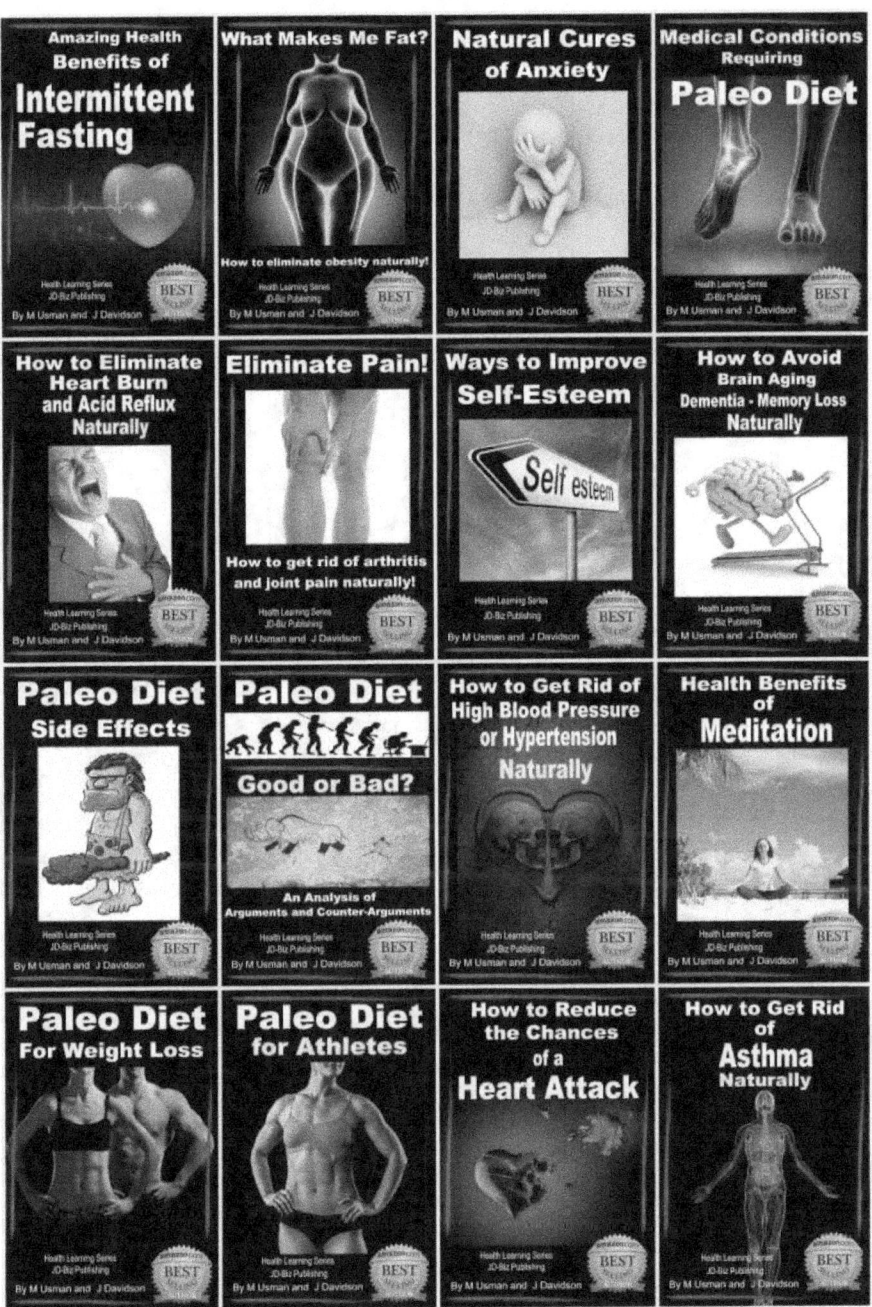

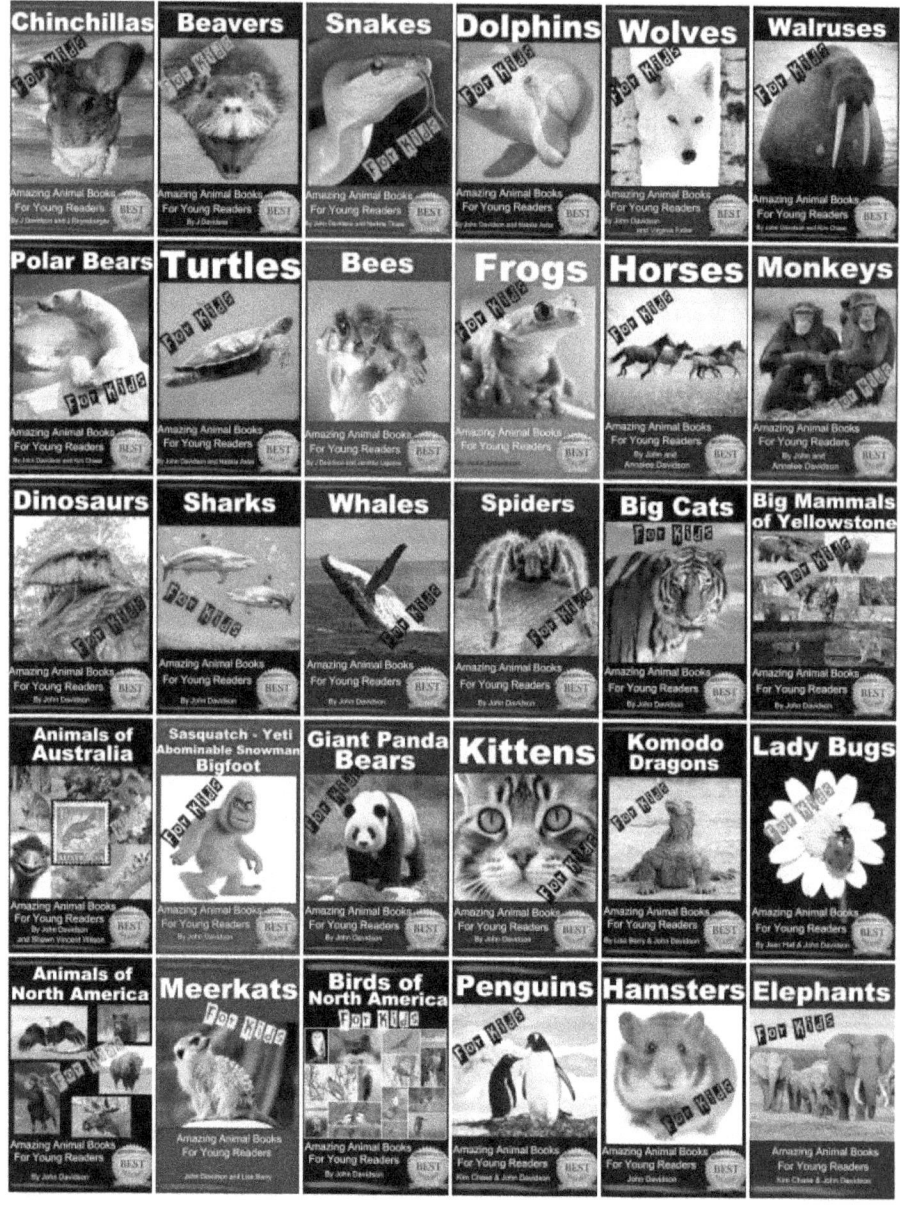

Learn To Draw Series

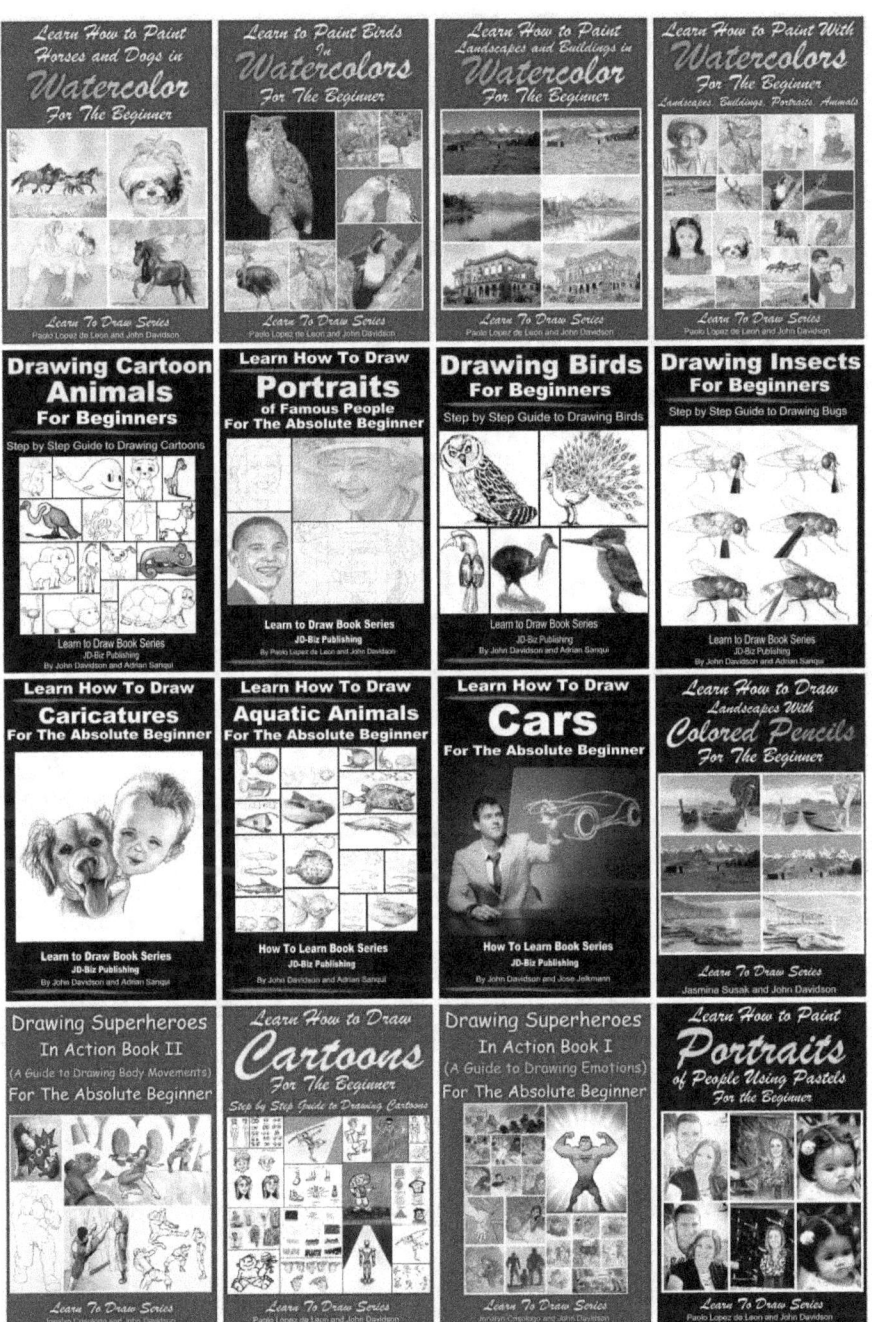

How to Build and Plan Books

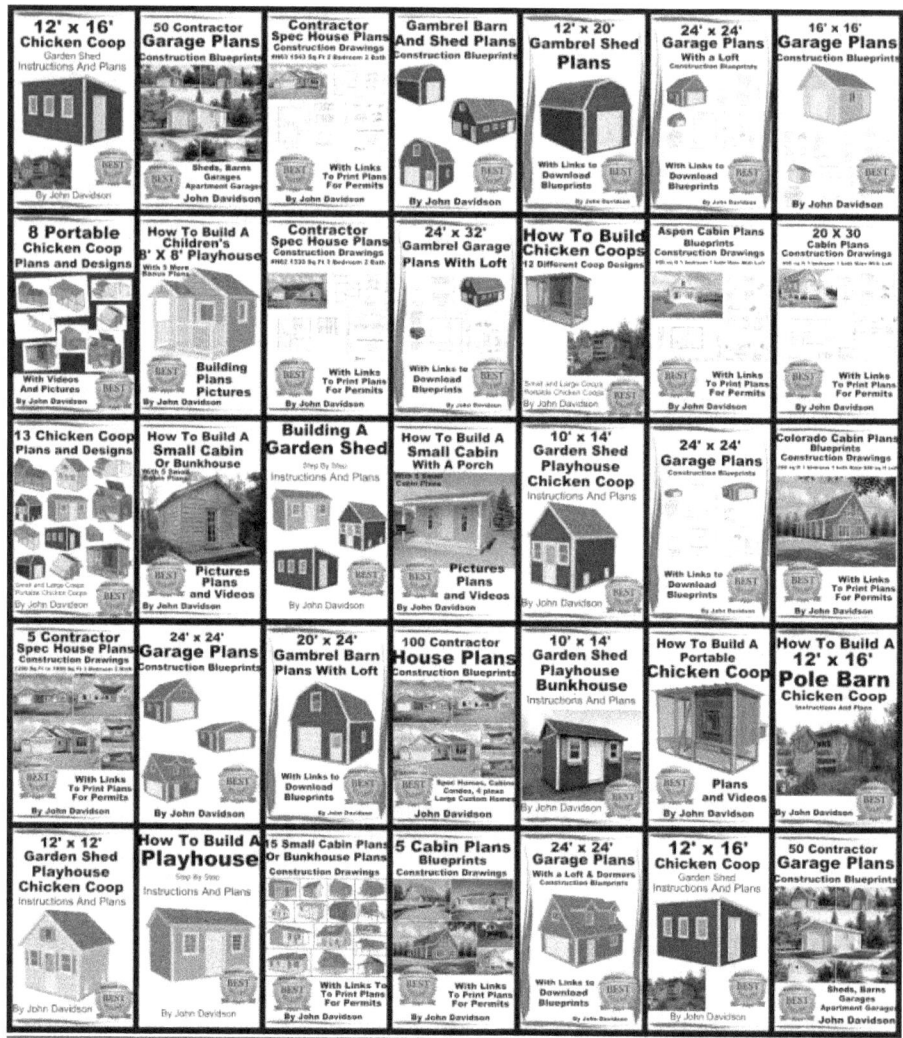

Entrepreneur Book Series

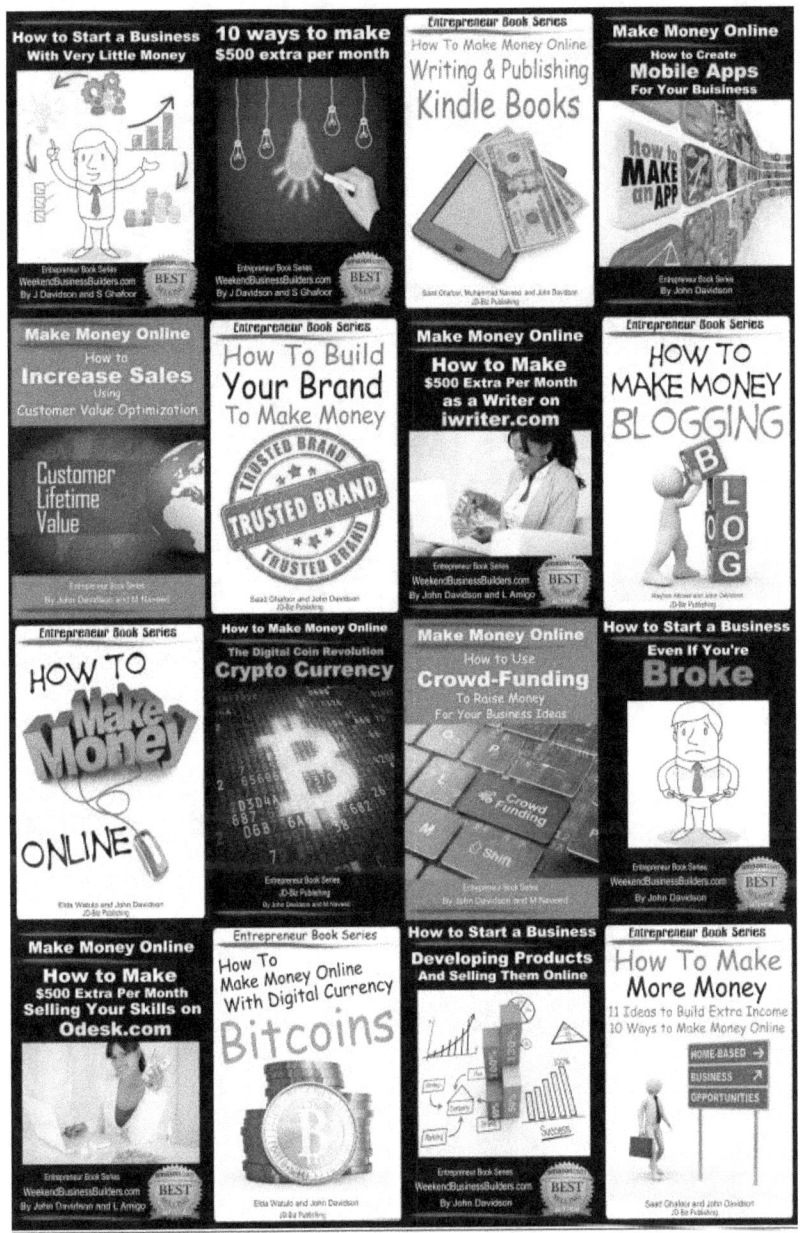

Our books are available at

1. Amazon.com

2. Barnes and Noble

3. Itunes

4. Kobo

5. Smashwords

6. Google Play Books

Publisher

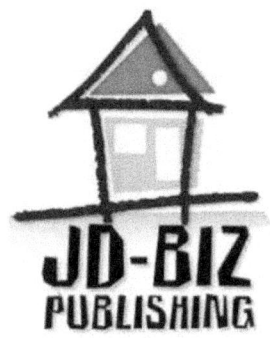

JD-Biz Corp

P O Box 374

Mendon, Utah 84325

http://www.jd-biz.com/

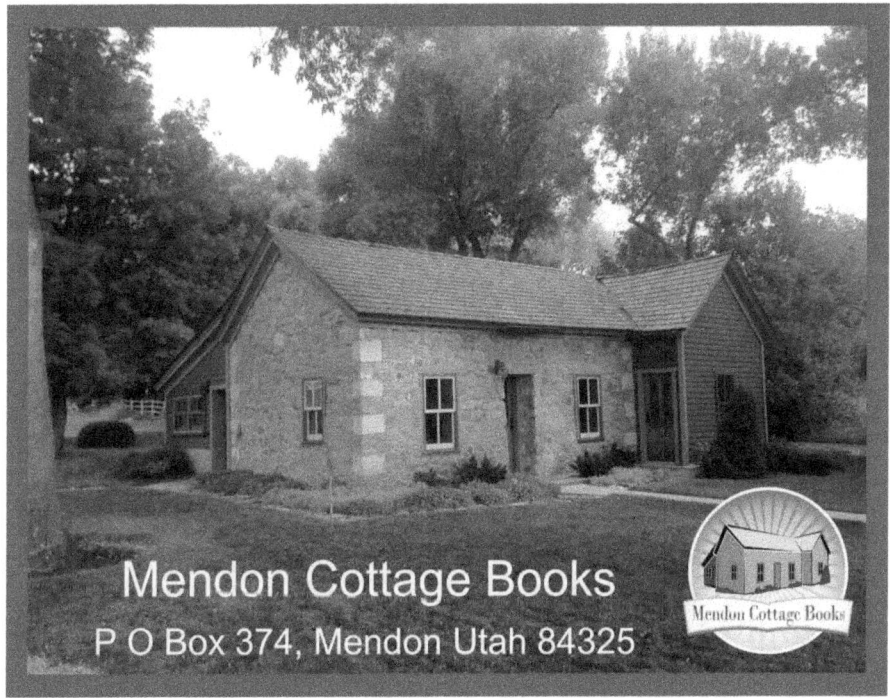

Mendon Cottage Books

P O Box 374, Mendon Utah 84325

www.ingramcontent.com/pod-product-compliance
Lightning Source LLC
Chambersburg PA
CBHW070344290526
45791CB00003B/1466